NAVIGATING PROLAPSED UTERUS WITH CONFIDENCE AND CARE

Discovering Resilience And Empowering Solutions For Confronting Challenges For A Healthy Reproductive System

DR. WESLEY IAN

DISCLAIMER

The information in this book is not meant to replace professional medical advice, diagnosis, or treatment; rather, it is meant mainly for general informational reasons. If you have any questions about a medical problem, you should always consult your doctor or another trained health expert. Don't ever discount expert medical advice or put off getting it because of something you've read in this book.

Any negative effects or repercussions arising from the usage of the material provided herein are not the responsibility of the book's author or publisher. It should be noted by readers that the material in this book is not all-inclusive and might not address every facet of the subject. Furthermore, new research may have an impact on how health concerns are understood or treated because medical knowledge is always changing.

No particular test, treatment, method, or product mentioned in this book is endorsed or promoted by the author or publisher. The reader assumes all risk associated with using the information included in this book.

Before making any big decisions regarding your health, it's crucial to speak with a licensed healthcare provider. The relationship between a patient and their healthcare practitioner should not be replaced by this book, nor is it meant to offer medical advice.

The opinions presented in this book are the author's and may not necessarily represent those of the publisher. Any errors, omissions, or inaccuracies in the information in this book are not the responsibility of the author or publisher.

It is recommended that readers independently confirm any information contained in this book and speak with a healthcare provider about their specific medical needs and state of health.

TABLE OF CONTENTS

ABOUT THE BOOK

"Navigating Prolapsed Uterus with Confidence and Care" is an all-inclusive manual that covers all the complex aspects of a prolapsed uterus and provides vital information for patients and medical professionals who are involved in their care. Prolapsed uterus, a medical disorder when the uterus descends into or beyond the vaginal canal, is explored in detail in the book's enlightening introduction.

The book lay the groundwork by explaining the fundamentals of female anatomy, providing a thorough synopsis of the female reproductive system, and outlining the standard uterine position. The book then explores the critical topic of identifying symptoms and indications, advising readers on whether to seek medical assistance and how to proceed with the diagnostic process.

The several forms of uterine prolapsed, together with their underlying causes and risk factors, are described in great detail. Through an extensive examination of variables like aging, childbearing, pregnancy, and weak pelvic floor, the book offers a full knowledge of the illness.

The book devotes a large amount of its content to lifestyle changes, pelvic floor exercises, preventative tactics, safe lifting practices, and keeping a healthy weight. With the help of these useful tools, readers may either manage the progression of prolapsed or reduce its danger.

The book examines medical treatment options—both surgical and non-surgical—in the ensuing chapters, offering a fair assessment of the advantages and disadvantages of each. It also explores the lifestyle and emotional implications of having a prolapsed uterus, including advice on negotiating intimate relationships, coping mechanisms, and support systems.

The book offers specific information on how to manage prolapsed during pregnancy, address delivery alternatives, and provide postpartum care, acknowledging the particular difficulties that pregnant women with prolapsed uteruses confront.

Furthermore, the book, which covers lifestyle, nutrition, and alternative therapies, takes a comprehensive approach to care. Building self-esteem and confidence, as well as promoting self-care and empowerment through knowledge, are the main topics.

The book offers helpful tools and guidance to readers on how to locate trustworthy information, interact with communities and support groups, and seek professional help. "Navigating Prolapsed Uterus with Confidence and Care" is a priceless tool that combines medical knowledge with useful advice to improve the well-being of people navigating the challenges associated with a prolapsed uterus.

CHAPTER ONE

INTRODUCTION TO PROLAPSED UTERUS

COMPREHENDING UTERINE PROLAPSED

The organs that make up the human body are carefully constructed, complicated systems that are vital to the preservation of general health. The uterus is one such organ in the female reproductive system that is extremely important. A prolapsed uterus is one of the conditions that might cause the uterus to fail, even though it is a tough organ. The uterus descends or is displaced from its typical location within the pelvic cavity in this medical disorder. Investigating the definition, types, causes, and risk factors of a prolapsed uterus is necessary to comprehend its complexities.

DEFINITION

The uterus's downward displacement from its normal position within the pelvic cavity is the hallmark of a prolapsed uterus. Weakened pelvic floor muscles and ligaments that support the uterus may be the cause of this displacement. The uterus, bladder, and rectum are held in place by the pelvic floor, which functions as a sling. If these supporting components are damaged, the uterus may come out of the body in severe cases or sink into the vaginal canal. Pregnancy and childbirth are the main causes of a prolapsed uterus, though there are other variables as well. Uterine prolapsed may become more likely due to the stress of childbirth and the strain exerted on the pelvic floor during pregnancy, which can weaken the supporting tissues.

PROLAPSE TYPES

Understanding the varied manifestations of a prolapsed uterus is essential for a proper diagnosis and suitable therapy. The most prevalent kind is anterior prolapse, sometimes referred to as cystocele, in which the uterus's front wall descends into the vaginal canal. Rectocele, also known as posterior prolapse, is the result of the uterus's back wall pushing into the vaginal area. Furthermore, there are two types of uterine prolapse: total, in which the entire uterus descends into the vagina, and incomplete, in which only a part of the uterus protrudes. Every variety exhibits unique indications and can necessitate customized measures to tackle particular issues.

SYNOPSIS OF THE FEMALE REPRODUCTIVE SYSTEM

The female reproductive system is a sophisticated and multifaceted network of organs that is essential to the body's ability to reproduce and regulate its hormones. This system consists of several structures, each of which has a distinct role and adds to the overall reproduction process. The uterus, an organ with a pear shape that is located in the pelvic cavity, is one of the main parts of the female reproductive system.

THE STRUCTURE AND FUNCTION OF THE UTERUS

During pregnancy, the uterus acts as the growing fetus's gestational chamber. It is a muscular organ with an endometrial lining that changes cyclically in response to changes in hormone levels. The ovaries, which create, release, and, if conception does place, fertilize the eggs, are in charge of regulating these hormonal fluctuations. The fallopian tubes serve as passageways for the eggs as they go from the ovaries to the uterus, the site of fertilization.

The three primary layers that make up the uterine structure are the endometrium, which is the inner lining, the middle muscle layer called the myometrium, and the outermost serosa. The myometrium is very important during labor and delivery because the contractions help the baby come out of the uterus.

In reaction to hormonal cues, the endometrium goes through periodic modifications that get it ready for the possible implantation of a fertilized egg. The endometrial lining sheds during menstruation, signaling the start of a new menstrual cycle, if fertilization is unsuccessful. The health and fertility of a woman's reproductive system depend on this cyclical

CHAPTER TWO

UNDERSTANDING THE SYMPTOMS AND SIGNS

TYPICAL SIGNS OF UTERINE PROLAPSE INCLUDE

A prolapsed uterus is a disorder in which the uterus descends into the vaginal canal due to weakening of the pelvic muscles and ligaments supporting it. Identifying the symptoms and indicators is essential for prompt action. Pelvic pressure or fullness is one of the most typical signs of a prolapsed uterus. Some women report feeling as though something is dropping or bulging in the pelvic area. This pain could get worse when you lift heavy things, stand for long periods, or after giving birth.

Urinary problems are another common symptom. Urination frequency or urgency may rise in women who have a prolapsed uterus. Additionally, some people may experience involuntary pee leaks or trouble entirely emptying their bladder, particularly while engaging in activities that strain their pelvic floor. Additionally, uterine prolapse might manifest as sexual dysfunction. Women may experience pain or discomfort when having sex, and when they examine themselves, they may discover a bulge or protrusion.

WHEN TO GET MEDICAL HELP

Managing a prolapsed uterus effectively requires knowing when to seek medical assistance. A woman must get medical attention if she has ongoing pelvic pain, pressure, or discomfort. A trip to the gynecologist is recommended in the event of any discernible protrusion or bulging from the vaginal entrance. Women should seek immediate medical attention if they observe changes in their urine patterns, such as increased frequency, urgency, or trouble emptying the bladder.

Women who have recently given birth, especially those who delivered their child vaginally, should be on the lookout for any strange pelvic pain or symptoms. Seeking medical assistance as soon as possible facilitates a rapid diagnosis and intervention, both of which have a substantial impact on the course of treatment for uterine prolapse.

PROLAPSE DIAGNOSIS

A medical professional must perform a thorough examination to diagnose a prolapsed uterus. The pelvic examination entails the physician evaluating the position of the pelvic organs and documenting any obvious indications of prolapse. To provide a more thorough understanding of pelvic anatomy, further diagnostic procedures like magnetic resonance imaging (MRI) or ultrasound may be suggested in specific circumstances.

Healthcare professionals may employ a staging system, such as the Pelvic Organ Prolapse Quantification (POP-Q) system, to assess the degree of uterine prolapse. Treatment choices are guided by this method, which also aids in classifying the degree of organ descent. Assessing related symptoms, medical history, and other risk factors like age, past childbirth, and hormonal state are all part of the diagnostic procedure.

Prompt intervention depends on being aware of the warning signs and symptoms of a prolapsed uterus. To properly manage this illness, it is imperative to have a comprehensive diagnostic evaluation and know when to seek medical assistance. Women who have the right medical advice can explore

Many alternatives for treatment to deal with the symptoms and enhance their quality of life.

CHAPTER THREE

UTERINE PROLAPSE TYPES

A disorder known as uterine prolapse happens when the uterus descends into the vaginal canal as a result of weakening muscles and ligaments supporting it. Depending on the degree of descent, uterine prolapse severity is divided into several categories. These degrees aid in comprehending how the illness progresses and direct suitable therapy modalities.

FIRST-DEGREE PROLAPSE

The uterus descends very little in a first-degree uterine prolapse. The cervix does not protrude outside the vaginal opening, but it may descend into the vaginal canal. First-degree prolapse in women may be asymptomatic or produce only slight discomfort; they may not have any noticeable symptoms. Common conservative methods for controlling first-degree prolapse include pelvic floor exercises, lifestyle adjustments, and occasionally the use of pessaries, which are devices put into the vagina to give support.

SECOND-DEGREE PROLAPSE

In second-degree prolapse, the uterus descends into the vaginal canal more dramatically. When standing or straining—activities that raise intra-abdominal pressure—the cervix may at this stage extend slightly outside the vaginal opening. Back pain, discomfort during sexual activity, and a sensation of pressure in the pelvic area are among the symptoms that could become more apparent. For second-degree prolapse, pessary use, pelvic floor exercises, and conservative therapy are still effective choices; however, surgical intervention may be necessary in more severe cases.

THIRD-DEGREE PROLAPSE

Even during routine daily activities, the cervix protrudes outside the vaginal opening, indicating a considerable descent of the uterus. As the symptoms worsen, they could include constipation, trouble passing gas, and a noticeable protrusion in the vaginal region. To address the structural alterations and reestablish normal pelvic support, surgical intervention—such as uterine suspension or hysterectomy—may be advised. Conservative methods may only be able to provide minimal relief at this point.

COMPLETE PROLAPSE

The most severe type of uterine descent is complete uterine prolapse, sometimes referred to as procidentia. The entire uterus protrudes outside the vaginal opening in this situation. Prolapsed women may have significant symptoms, such as incontinence of the feces and urine, persistent pelvic pain, and difficulty walking.

To rectify the prolapse and give the pelvic organs the proper support, surgery is frequently required. To restore pelvic structure and function, treatments such as uterosacral ligament suspension and sacrocolpopexy may be used.

The categorization of uterine prolapse into varying degrees facilitates healthcare practitioners in customizing treatment plans according to the severity of the ailment. Depending on the degree of decline and the effect of symptoms on the patient's quality of life, conservative therapy or surgical intervention may be chosen. Accurate diagnosis and suitable management of uterine prolapse require routine pelvic exams and consultations with medical professionals.

CHAPTER FOUR

REASONS AND DANGER ELEMENTS
BEING PREGNANT AND GIVING BIRTH

A woman's health and well-being can be significantly impacted by pregnancy and childbirth. Numerous body systems may be under stress as a result of the physiological changes that occur during pregnancy, such as the uterus' growth and changes in hormone levels. Furthermore, the act of giving birth itself may cause stress to the pelvic area, which may weaken the pelvic floor muscles. These muscles are vital for maintaining the pelvic organs, and vaginal deliveries in particular may cause them to stretch and weaken.

MENOPAUSE AND AGING

Menopause and aging are normal life stages that can affect a person's chance of developing certain illnesses, such as pelvic floor diseases. Reduced muscle tone and tissue elasticity in women can be caused by hormonal changes, such as the drop in estrogen levels after menopause. Women may be more vulnerable to problems like pelvic organ prolapse and urine incontinence as a result of this physiological change that weakens the pelvic floor muscles. Pelvic floor dysfunction is more likely as a result of aging's effects on the connective tissues supporting the pelvic organs.

WEAKNESS IN THE PELVIC FLOOR

One of the main contributing factors to the development of pelvic floor problems is pelvic floor weakness. These muscles give the rectum, uterus, and bladder the vital support they need. Pelvic floor weakening can be brought on by several factors, including aging, delivery, and pregnancy. Apart from these main causes, lifestyle decisions like hard lifting, persistent coughing, and excessive straining during bowel movements can also lead to a decline in pelvic floor strength. Pelvic floor weakness can also be exacerbated by certain medical problems, such as obesity and persistent constipation, which increases the likelihood of pelvic floor diseases.

ADDITIONAL CONTRIBUTING ELEMENTS

There is a wide range of other contributing factors that can affect pelvic floor health. Genetics are involved, since those with a family history of pelvic floor problems may be more vulnerable.

Neurological diseases and other long-term medical issues can potentially affect pelvic floor function. Lifestyle choices that may impact blood circulation and general muscle tone, such as smoking and a sedentary way of living, can also lead to poor pelvic floor health. Moreover, traumas or procedures that directly impact the pelvic area may compromise the integrity of the pelvic floor and raise the possibility of dysfunction.

Realizing the complex interactions between many components is essential to gaining a thorough understanding of the causes and risk factors related to pelvic floor illnesses. Pelvic floor weakening, aging and menopause, pregnancy and childbirth, and a host of other events all contribute to the complex picture of pelvic floor health.

CHAPTER FIVE

PREVENTIVE TECHNIQUES

PELVIC FLOOR EXERCISES

Exercises for the pelvic floor are essential for preventative medicine, especially when it comes to women's health. These workouts focus on the muscles that support the uterus, rectum, and bladder, among other pelvic organs. Maintaining muscular tone and avoiding pelvic floor problems including prolapsed pelvic organs and urine incontinence require frequent pelvic floor training. These exercises are a great addition to any routine for women, especially those who have just given birth. Exercises for the pelvic floor, sometimes referred to as Kegel exercises, work the pelvic floor muscles by contracting and relaxing them to increase resilience and strength.

CHANGES IN LIFESTYLE

Lifestyle changes are essential to general health and well-being and play a major role in preventive measures. Making decisions that have a beneficial effect on one's physical and mental health is a necessary part of leading a healthy lifestyle. This includes eating well-balanced, nutrient-dense food, exercising frequently, controlling stress, and abstaining from bad habits like smoking and binge drinking.

These adjustments not only promote overall health but also help avoid several illnesses, including pelvic floor disorders. Leading a healthy lifestyle will help you maintain an ideal body weight and lower your risk of pelvic disorders linked to obesity.

THE RIGHT LIFTING METHODS

To avoid strain and injury on the pelvic floor and other musculoskeletal tissues, proper lifting techniques are crucial. The pelvic floor muscles may be overstressed by improper lifting techniques, which may lead to problems including pelvic organ prolapse.

People ought to be made aware of the value of bending at the knees, maintaining a straight back, and lifting heavy objects with their legs. It's important to avoid jerky, abrupt movements when lifting, and to distribute the weight evenly to reduce pressure on particular muscle areas, such as the pelvic region.

SUSTAINING A HEALTHY WEIGHT

A key component of preventing many health problems, including pelvic floor disorders, is maintaining a healthy weight. Being overweight increases the risk of pelvic floor problems by putting extra strain on the pelvic organs and supporting systems. The two most important things in managing weight are eating a balanced diet and exercising frequently.

Retaining a healthy weight benefits general health by lowering the risk of chronic diseases like diabetes, cardiovascular disease, and some types of cancer. It also helps prevent pelvic floor problems. Strategies for managing weight should be tailored to each person's needs and medical circumstances to support a long-term, comprehensive approach to well-being.

A comprehensive strategy for prevention entails focused training, dietary adjustments, safe lifting methods, and upholding a healthy weight. All of these techniques improve people's general health, but they are especially important in preventing pelvic floor diseases and their related repercussions. By enhancing longevity and quality of life, incorporating these behaviors into daily living can have a significant impact on health outcomes.

CHAPTER SIX

OPTIONS FOR MEDICAL TREATMENT

NONSURGICAL METHODS

In the field of medicine, non-surgical methods are vital since they provide an alternative to invasive surgeries and treatments. Physical therapy is a valuable and adaptable approach that can be used to treat a wide range of medical issues. Exercises, stretches, and manual treatments are used in physical therapy to increase function, reduce discomfort, and improve mobility. It is especially helpful for people who are trying to improve their musculoskeletal health, manage chronic diseases, or recuperate from injuries.

PHYSICAL MEDICINE

A vast array of interventions aimed at preserving, enhancing, and restoring the best possible physical function and quality of life are included in physical therapy. Licensed physical therapists create individualized treatment programs after assessing each patient's particular needs. Therapeutic activities to build muscle, increase flexibility, and improve coordination may be part of these regimens. To control pain and inflammation, physical therapists also use modalities like heat, cold, ultrasound, and electrical stimulation.

Physical therapy offers targeted therapies that often result in relief and increased functionality for patients with orthopedic difficulties, neurological disorders, or musculoskeletal injuries.

In addition, physical therapy is an essential component of prehabilitation, helping patients gets ready for impending procedures to improve their results thereafter. It is a crucial component of all-encompassing healthcare since it encourages both injury rehabilitation and proactive steps to lower the chance of developing new health problems.

Physical therapy's collaborative character, which involves the patient and the therapist, encourages a proactive approach to health and wellbeing.

PESSARIES

Another non-surgical approach for treating specific medical issues, mostly those associated with abnormalities of the pelvic floor, is pessaries.

 By being put into the vagina, these medical devices are intended to support the pelvic organs, such as the bladder or uterus. Because pessaries are available in a variety of sizes and shapes, medical experts can select the one that best suits a patient's medical demands and anatomical requirements.

Pelvic organ prolapse is a disorder where the pelvic organs fall into the vaginal space as a result of weakening pelvic floor muscles. One of the main uses of pessaries is in the management of this ailment.

To relieve symptoms such as pelvic pressure, urine incontinence, and pain, pessaries provide support to these structures. Additionally, by supporting the bladder neck, pessaries can be used to treat stress urine incontinence.

Because it is a conservative and reversible method, pessary use is a good choice for women who would want to postpone or avoid surgery. It is vital to schedule routine follow-up sessions with healthcare specialists to guarantee appropriate fitting, comfort, and upkeep of the prosthesis.

This non-invasive technique emphasizes the value of tailored care when choosing the right interventions, taking patient preferences, lifestyle, and medical history into account.

SURGICAL SOLUTIONS

Surgical interventions are vital to the medical industry because they provide effective relief from a wide range of ailments. These operations are frequently advised when more urgent and significant intervention is required or when non-surgical therapies prove to be ineffective. Surgical options vary widely, depending on the type and severity of the medical ailment. They include minimally invasive techniques as well as sophisticated surgeries.

SURGICAL PROCEDURE TYPES

Numerous surgical techniques are available that are expertly and precisely tailored to address particular health conditions. Smaller incisions and cutting-edge equipment are used in minimally invasive operations, such as laparoscopy and arthroscopy, to access and treat internal organs or structures. Comparing these techniques to open operations, the usual outcome is less pain following surgery, quicker recovery, and less scarring.

Major surgical procedures, on the other hand, require wider incisions that provide doctors with direct access to the damaged areas. In severe circumstances like organ transplants, open heart surgery, or large tumor removals, these procedures are required. This also includes elective procedures like cosmetic surgery, which are intended to improve appearance and increase patient confidence.

Surgeon skills and cutting-edge technology are combined in robotic-assisted procedures. Robotic systems are controlled by surgeons to carry out complex operations with improved dexterity and less invasiveness. This method offers better visibility and flexibility in small locations, making it especially useful for delicate surgeries.

PERILS AND ADVANTAGES

Surgical operations have inherent hazards as well as potential advantages, just like any other medical intervention. Infection, hemorrhages, anesthesia-related side effects, and occasionally harm to the surrounding tissues or organs are among the dangers associated with surgery. The degree of these hazards is determined by several variables, including the surgeon's experience, the intricacy of the procedure, and the general health of the patient.

On the other hand, surgical operations can have significant positive effects by offering a long-term reprieve from or a solution to medical problems. In addition to treating anatomical defects and relieving chronic pain, surgery can greatly enhance a patient's quality of life. Minimally invasive procedures frequently result in quick recovery and a return to regular daily activities, which adds to the overall beneficial effect on patients' well-being.

In addition, the choice to have surgery requires serious evaluation of the advantages and disadvantages. To obtain informed consent, patients and healthcare professionals have in-depth conversations that enable people to balance the benefits of the intervention against any possible drawbacks. Collaboration between patients, surgeons, and the larger healthcare team is often essential to the success of surgical results to maximize preoperative planning and aftercare.

COPING MECHANISMS FOR A PROLAPSED UTERUS

Living with a prolapsed uterus can be difficult, requiring people to manage many emotional and physical facets of their health. Coping mechanisms are essential for handling the day-to-day difficulties brought on by this illness. Getting expert advice from medical professionals who specialize in women's health is one successful strategy. These experts can provide customized guidance on exercises, dietary changes, and other tactics to reduce discomfort and improve general pelvic health.

PSYCHOLOGICAL WELLNESS

Living with a prolapsed uterus involves many aspects, one of which is emotional well-being. Recognizing and treating any arising frustration, anxiety, or despair is essential to managing the emotional effects of a prolapse. Seeking assistance from mental health specialists, such as counselors or therapists, can offer a secure environment for managing and exploring these feelings. Joining online forums or support groups where people exchange stories can also help people feel more connected and understanding.

ASSISTANCE NETWORKS

Support systems are essential for assisting people in overcoming the difficulties associated with a prolapsed uterus. A supportive environment can be created by being open and honest about the disease with friends and family. People can handle their everyday lives more easily when they get empathy, emotional support, and practical help from loved ones. In certain situations, including a spouse in the choices made about lifestyle modifications and treatment alternatives might fortify the support system.

MODIFICATIONS TO LIFESTYLE

Living with a prolapsed uterus often requires modifying one's lifestyle. Exercises that are low-impact and often prescribed by medical specialists can assist in strengthening the pelvic floor muscles and reduce discomfort. Maintaining a healthy weight and eating a balanced diet are also vital components of a healthy lifestyle that can enhance general well-being. People may need to adjust their daily routines to prevent strenuous lifting and high-impact exercises that can make their prolapse worse.

Managing a prolapsed uterus necessitates a holistic strategy that takes into account both the mental and physical facets of well-being. Developing a solid support system and obtaining competent assistance are two crucial coping mechanisms for chronic illness. It is important to prioritize emotional well-being, and people are advised to check into mental health services to deal with any emotional difficulties that may come up. A balanced diet and regular exercise are two important lifestyle changes that can help improve the quality of life for people who have a prolapsed uterus.

CHAPTER SEVEN

HANDLING CLOSE RELATIONSHIPS

SPEAKING WITH YOUR SPOUSE

A strong and happy personal connection is built on effective communication. It entails attentively listening to your spouse as well as expressing your ideas and feelings. In addition to fostering understanding and establishing trust, open and honest communication also fortifies the emotional bond between partners. Establishing a secure environment in which both parties can freely express their opinions without worrying about criticism is essential. Active listening, confirming your partner's emotions, and showing empathy for their viewpoint are all necessary for this.

To navigate personal relationships, it's critical to share both your good and bad experiences. A happy environment can be created by expressing love, thanks, and appreciation; conversing about issues, disagreements, or unfulfilled needs facilitates development and resolution. Setting limits and being explicit about expectations are other important aspects of healthy communication that guarantee that both parties understand the dynamics of the partnership.

TAKING CARE OF SEXUAL PROBLEMS

Keeping a satisfying connection requires taking care of sexual problems, which are an important part of many romantic partnerships. To make sure that both partners are at ease and content, an honest discussion about preferences, boundaries, and aspirations is crucial. When it comes to sexual intimacy, people may have various wants and expectations, so it's critical to acknowledge this and create a middle ground that respects each person's desires.

Discussing preferences, trying out novel behaviors, and, if necessary, obtaining professional assistance are some ways to address sexual difficulties. Respecting each other's body language and emotions is essential to a fulfilling sexual connection. Moreover, a strong sexual connection requires an atmosphere in which both partners feel comfortable talking about their wants and worries without fear of rejection or embarrassment.

LOOKING FOR EXPERT ADVICE

Occasionally, managing close connections could necessitate consulting a specialist. Relationship therapy or counseling can provide insightful information and useful techniques for resolving issues, enhancing communication, and fortifying the bond overall. Expert advice offers an unbiased viewpoint, enabling both parties to discuss their worries in a controlled and encouraging setting.

When dealing with enduring problems like communication breakdowns, trust concerns, or sexual challenges, counseling can be especially helpful. A qualified therapist can assist in seeing behavioral patterns, encouraging candid conversation, and assisting couples in moving toward a more positive dynamic. Seeking expert advice is a proactive step toward developing a strong and satisfying relationship rather than a show of weakness. It exhibits a dedication to interpersonal and personal development, building a basis for contentment and enjoyment over the long run.

CHAPTER EIGHT

PROLAPSE AND PREGNANCY

TAKING CARE OF PROLAPSE DURING GESTATION

Pelvic floor muscles and ligaments can weaken during pregnancy, causing the uterus, bladder, or rectum to descend into the vaginal canal. This condition is known as pelvic organ prolapse. Pregnancy-related prolapse management calls for an all-encompassing strategy that addresses the particular difficulties and factors involved with this condition.

Pelvic floor exercises are a vital component of controlling prolapse during pregnancy. By strengthening the pelvic floor muscles, these exercises—often referred to as Kegels—hope to improve pelvic organ support.

It is important to teach women the correct form for doing Kegel exercises and to motivate them to do so regularly. It's crucial to remember that not every woman can perform every exercise and that getting personalized advice from medical professionals is crucial.

DELIVERY CHOICES

Options for delivery are important when it comes to managing prolapse throughout pregnancy. For women with mild to severe prolapse, vaginal delivery is typically regarded as safe, as long as the medical team keeps a constant eye on the patient.

To lessen the possibility of further harm to the pelvic floor, a cesarean section could be advised in situations with severe prolapse or difficulties.

The woman and her healthcare professional should work together to decide on the delivery method, taking into consideration the particulars of her prolapse and general health.

To support women in their recovery and address any remaining difficulties, postpartum care is an essential element of managing prolapse.

For women with prolapse, pelvic floor rehabilitation—which consists of focused exercises and physical therapy—is an essential element of postpartum treatment? Guidance on gradually returning to normal activities and avoiding activities that could strain the pelvic floor should be given by healthcare providers.

AFTERPARTUM CARE

Regular follow-up visits are also essential as part of postpartum care to monitor the development of pelvic organ prolapse and handle any potential issues or complications.

For women to seek immediate medical assistance when necessary, they should be informed about the warning signs and symptoms of increasing prolapse, such as increased pelvic pressure or bulging sensations.

During this time, women may suffer anxiety or worry about their general well-being and pelvic health, so emotional support is also essential.

To summarize, the management of prolapse during pregnancy necessitates a comprehensive strategy that includes pelvic floor exercises, thoughtful deliberation about delivery alternatives, and thorough postpartum care.

Through coordinated efforts with healthcare providers, women can manage pregnancy and childbirth while prioritizing the preservation and restoration of their pelvic health.

CHAPTER NINE

MATERIALS AND ASSISTANCE

LOCATING TRUSTED INFORMATION

One of the most important skills for traversing the wide terrain of knowledge available today is finding trustworthy information. It is getting harder and harder to tell which sources are genuine and which are not, especially with the abundance of information available online. When looking for information, it's important to use judgment and critical thinking while taking the reliability, correctness, and relevance of the sources into account.

Reputable organizations, subject-matter specialists, or peer-reviewed publications are frequently sources of trustworthy information. A comprehensive and precise grasp of a subject can be ensured by fact-checking and cross-referencing information from other sources, which can further improve the information's credibility.

COMMUNITIES AND SUPPORT GROUPS

Communities and support networks are essential for giving people a feeling of acceptance and comprehension. These groups serve a variety of interests, needs, and challenges and are available both online and offline. Whether dealing with health problems, changes in lifestyle, or personal challenges, joining a support group can provide emotional support, a forum for sharing experiences, and insightful information. Social media groups and forums on the internet have made it easier to create virtual communities where people from all over the world can connect and support one another. Joining these groups helps to build a sense of community by dismantling obstacles to isolation and establishing a forum for support and encouragement from one another.

EXPERT SUPPORT

People frequently turn to professionals for help when they face difficulties that need certain knowledge, abilities, or competence. This can entail consulting experts like physicians, attorneys, therapists, or financial consultants. Getting professional help guarantees that people have access to specialized, research-backed solutions that give them knowledgeable support for their particular requirements. Seeking professional assistance—whether in the form of therapeutic interventions, legal counsel, or medical advice—is a proactive step in developing workable solutions and accomplishing desired results. Professionals give individualized solutions and advice to tackle challenging circumstances because of their depth of knowledge and expertise.

Obtaining trustworthy information, interacting with communities and support networks, and seeking professional help are all integral parts of a comprehensive strategy for promoting individual and societal well-being.

The capacity to recognize reliable information is essential in the digital era, and organizations and groups can offer emotional and community support that can be a source of strength. Moreover, consulting a professional guarantees access to specific knowledge and experience, empowering people to tackle obstacles with assurance and effectiveness. When combined, these ideas provide a solid basis for wise choices, individual development, and a nurturing social circle.